Acting Edition

Uncle Vanya

Scenes from a Country Life in Four Acts

adapted by Heidi Schreck

based on a co-translation by Tatyana Khaikin and Heidi Schreck

from Anton Chekhov

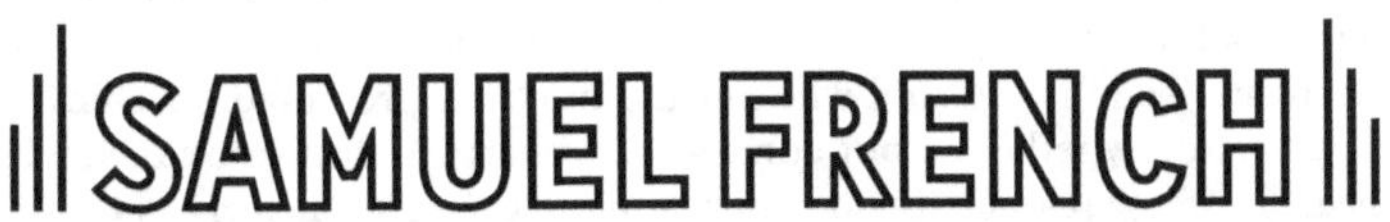

Copyright © 2025 by Heidi Schreck
Cover image: *Sonya Brings Tea*
Copyright © 2007 by Deirdre O'Connell
Used with permission.
All Rights Reserved

UNCLE VANYA is fully protected under the copyright laws of the United States of America, the British Commonwealth, including Canada, and all member countries of the Berne Convention for the Protection of Literary and Artistic Works, the Universal Copyright Convention, and/or the World Trade Organization conforming to the Agreement on Trade Related Aspects of Intellectual Property Rights. All rights, including professional and amateur stage productions, recitation, lecturing, public reading, motion picture, radio broadcasting, television, online/digital production, and the rights of translation into foreign languages are strictly reserved.

ISBN 978-0-573-71163-3

www.concordtheatricals.com
www.concordtheatricals.co.uk

FOR PRODUCTION INQUIRIES

UNITED STATES AND CANADA
info@concordtheatricals.com
1-866-979-0447

UNITED KINGDOM AND EUROPE
licensing@concordtheatricals.co.uk
020-7054-7298

Each title is subject to availability from Concord Theatricals Corp., depending upon country of performance. Please be aware that *UNCLE VANYA* may not be licensed by Concord Theatricals Corp. in your territory. Professional and amateur producers should contact the nearest Concord Theatricals Corp. office or licensing partner to verify availability.

CAUTION: Professional and amateur producers are hereby warned that *UNCLE VANYA* is subject to a licensing fee. The purchase, renting, lending or use of this book does not constitute a license to perform this title(s), which license must be obtained from Concord Theatricals Corp. prior to any performance. Performance of this title(s) without a license is a violation of federal law and may subject the producer and/or presenter of such performances to civil penalties. Both amateurs and professionals considering a production are strongly advised to apply to the appropriate agent before starting rehearsals, advertising, or booking a theatre. A licensing fee must be paid whether the title(s) is presented for charity or gain and whether or not admission is charged. Professional/Stock licensing fees are quoted upon application to Concord Theatricals Corp.

This work is published by Samuel French, an imprint of Concord Theatricals Corp.

No one shall make any changes in this title(s) for the purpose of production. No part of this book may be reproduced, stored in a retrieval system, scanned, uploaded, or transmitted in any form, by any means, now known or yet to be invented, including mechanical, electronic, digital, photocopying, recording, videotaping, or otherwise, without the prior written permission of the publisher. No one shall share this title(s), or any part of this title(s), through any social media or file hosting websites.

For all inquiries regarding motion picture, television, online/digital and other media rights, please contact Concord Theatricals Corp.

MUSIC AND THIRD-PARTY MATERIALS USE NOTE

Licensees are solely responsible for obtaining formal written permission from copyright owners to use copyrighted music and/or other copyrighted third-party materials (e.g. artworks, logos) in the performance of this play and are strongly cautioned to do so. If no such permission is obtained by the licensee, then the licensee must use only original music and materials that the licensee owns and controls. Licensees are solely responsible and liable for clearances of all third-party copyrighted materials, including without limitation music, and shall indemnify the copyright owners of the play(s) and their licensing agent, Concord Theatricals Corp., against any costs, expenses, losses and liabilities arising from the use of such copyrighted third-party materials by licensees. For music, please contact the appropriate music licensing authority in your territory for the rights to any incidental music.

IMPORTANT BILLING AND CREDIT REQUIREMENTS

If you have obtained performance rights to this title, please refer to your licensing agreement for important billing and credit requirements.

UNCLE VANYA was first produced by Lincoln Center Theater (André Bishop, Producing Artistic Director; Adam Siegel, Managing Director) and premiered at the Vivian Beaumont Theater in New York City on April 24, 2024. The production was directed by Lila Neugebauer, with sets by Mimi Lien, costumes by Kaye Voyce, lighting by Lap Chi Chu and Elizabeth Harper, and sound by Mikhail Fiksel and Beth Lake. The assistant to the playwright was Molly Paige, and the dramaturg was Jenna Clark Embrey. The associate director was Caitlin Ryan O'Connell and the production stage manager was Charles M. Turner III. The cast was as follows:

PROFESSOR ALEXANDER	Alfred Molina
YELENA	Anika Noni Rose
SONYA	Alison Pill
MARIA	Jayne Houdyshell
VANYA	Steve Carell
ASTROV	William Jackson Harper
WAFFLES	Jonathan Hadary
MARINA	Mia Katigbak
NEIGHBOR	Spencer Donovan Jones

CHARACTERS

PROFESSOR ALEXANDER – a retired professor

YELENA – his wife

SONYA – his daughter by his first marriage

MARIA – a local politician's widow and mother of the professor's first wife

VANYA – her son

ASTROV – a doctor

WAFFLES – a family friend

MARINA – Sonya's childhood nanny

NEIGHBOR – a local kid

SETTING

The action takes place on the family's country estate, a working farm.

AUTHOR'S NOTE

When I agreed to create a new translation of *Uncle Vanya* for Lincoln Center, my dream was to remain as faithful as possible to the text while allowing the language to feel immediate, alive, and unmistakably American. Director Lila Neugebauer envisioned a contemporary staging that didn't announce its contemporariness; instead, she wanted the story to feel effortlessly rooted in the "here-and-now," to unfold in a world shaped by economic precarity, threatened by climate destruction, and haunted by our own questions about life's purpose, love, and the value of our labor.

To serve this vision, I approached the work as a kind of "quiet" adaptation rather than a bold re-imagining. I wanted to listen closely to the play and gently shift its context, asking: What happens when a Russian masterpiece about disillusionment and desire is filtered through the particular disillusionments of our own time and place? What does it feel like to hear these characters speak in a familiar cadence? To watch them navigate a world shaped by not by czarist Russia but by American late-stage capitalism and the despair and spiritual fatigue we live with right now? What might it feel like to erase the distance between now and then, us and them?

I'm grateful to my brilliant co-translator, Tatyana Khaikin, for the countless hours she spent helping me untangle archaic idioms and incredibly long sentences, and for consistently anchoring me in Chekhov's expansive humor and compassion. And, of course, I'm thankful to Anton Chekhov himself, who understood that the ache to be useful, to be loved, and to forge meaning from our lives – however small – is eternal, and who also reminds us, over and over in both his stories and plays, that "life is given to us only once."

SPECIAL THANKS

Ayanna Thompson, Kate Wilson, Julia Judge, Jessica Niebanck, Laura Stuart, James R. Geoghegan, Paul Smithyman, Kevin Orzechowski, Polina Minchuk Macklin, Sarah Azizo, Matthew Markoff, Mia Rosenfeld, Christopher Rungoo, Brittany Vasta, Amanda Gladu, Tommy Kurzman, Nikiya Mathis, Alexander Le Vaillant Freer, Edward S. Hansen, Noel Nichols, Megan Culley, Alex Wylie, Olive Barrett, Kaitlin Leigh Marsh, Monét Thibou, Matthew Pezzulich, Michael Bryan French, Marceline Hugot, Brenda Meaney, Stephen Conrad Moore, Robert Stanton, Naomi Grabel, Karin Schall, Maggie Greene, Sarah Marlin, Linda Mason Ross, Julia Stevens, Jenny Loeffler, Mimi Rios, Rheba Flegelman, Juliana Hannett, Nick Buchholz, Mala Mosher, Meghan Lantzy, William Nagle, Joe DiFonzo, Keith Schnacke, John Weingart, Kyle Barrineau, Charlie Rausenberger, Will Sweeney, Margaret Lazenby, Kathleen Gallagher, Susie Ghebresillassie, Barry Hoff, Mark Trezza, Natalia Castilla, Bruce Rubin, Kevin Johnson, Michael Bert, Charles Shell, Bridget O'Conner, Mark Parenti, Kip Fagan, Alex Barron, Bathsheba Doran, Lili Fagan-Schreck, Frankie Fagan-Schreck, Quincy Bernstine, Aaron Fili, Deirdre O'Connell, Maria Striar, Rachel Viola

ACT ONE

(A garden. A house with a terrace is visible in the distance. In an avenue of trees, under an old poplar, a table is set for lunch.)

*(***MARINA***, an unhurried older woman, sits at the table. ***ASTROV*** paces.)*

MARINA. Eat something, sweetie.

ASTROV. I don't feel like it.

MARINA. How about a little drink?

ASTROV. No. I don't drink every day. Besides, it's too muggy.

(Pause.)

Marina, how long have we known each other?

MARINA. *(Thinking.)* How long? Dear God. You moved out here...when? Sonya's mama was still alive. You were taking care of her for two years before she died. So that's...what? Eleven years already. *(She thinks.)* Maybe more...

ASTROV. Have I changed much?

MARINA. So much. You were young and handsome then and now you're old. Not so handsome. And I have to say, you do like your booze.

ASTROV. Yep... In ten years I've become a different person. You know why? I work too much, Marina. I'm on my feet all day, I don't get any rest, and at night I lie awake terrified, waiting for the next patient to drag me out of bed. I haven't had a day off the whole time we've known each other. Of course I got old! And life out here is stupid, boring, dirty… it chews you up. We're surrounded by freaks, nothing but freaks. Spend a few years out here and, little by little, you turn into a freak yourself.

(**ASTROV** *plays with his mustache.*)

Look, a huge mustache has sprouted up on my face – what a stupid mustache! I've turned into a freak. I'm not an idiot thank God – not yet – I've still got a brain in my head, but I feel numb. I don't want anything, I don't need anything, I don't love anybody. Well, you, maybe, are the only person I love.

(*He kisses her on the head.*)

MARINA. You should eat something.

ASTROV. Noooooo. In March, I had to go into town because of that flu outbreak. *(Beat.)* The clinic was crammed with people… families packed into the hallways… little kids… old folks lying on the floors. The smell…

(*Pause.*)

I ran from patient to patient all day, didn't sit down, didn't have a single bite to eat, and when I finally made it home, they still wouldn't let me rest! Some guy from the railroad was hit – a young guy – so they call me back in and when I try to patch him up, he goes and dies on me under anesthesia. And right then, when I didn't need them, all my feelings came rushing back. It felt like something was…*stabbing* at my conscience, as if I'd killed him on purpose… *(Beat.)* I sat down, closed my eyes – like this – and thought: the people who are alive a hundred years from now, two hundred years – what will they think of us? Will they remember us with kindness? Marina, they won't.

MARINA. People won't, but God will.

ASTROV. Ha, thank you. Those are nice words.

> (**VANYA** *enters from the house. He looks a bit rumpled.*)

VANYA. Yeah...

> (*Pause.*)

Yeah...

ASTROV. Nice nap?

VANYA. Yeah...what a nap. (*Yawns.*) Since the professor showed up with his *spouse*, my life has been chaos. I sleep at weird times, eat spicy food, drink wine all day... it's so unhealthy! Sonya and I used to do nothing but work all day! And now she's doing everything by herself, and I just eat, sleep, and drink myself stupid. Not good!

MARINA. It's chaos! The professor snoozes till noon, and we have to wait around for him to get up before we can have breakfast. We used to eat dinner at five o'clock like decent people, now it's not till seven. Then he stays up all night working, and at two in the morning, all of a sudden decides to ring his little bell. "What is it sweet man?" "I'm hungry!" So *somebody* has to get up and fix him a snack. (*Beat.*) Chaos!

ASTROV. How long are they staying?

VANYA. (*Whistling.*) A hundred years. The professor has decided to *live amongst the people.*

MARINA. Look! Lunch has been on the table for two hours and they're still out taking a walk!

PROFESSOR. (*Offstage.*) Beautiful, beautiful...

VANYA. They're coming, they're coming, don't panic.

(Voices. The **PROFESSOR**, **YELENA**, **SONYA**, *and* **WAFFLES** *emerge from the garden, back from their stroll.)*

PROFESSOR. Astonishing scenery! The views are magnificent.

WAFFLES. Yes indeed, Professor. Sir. Miraculous!

SONYA. Tomorrow we can take you out to see the forest, Dad. Would you like that?

VANYA. Ladies and gentlemen, lunch is served!

PROFESSOR. My friends, I'll take lunch in my office today if you don't mind! Have someone bring it in to me.

SONYA. You're going to love the forest, Dad...

*(***YELENA**, **PROFESSOR**, *and* **SONYA** *exit into the house.* **WAFFLES** *sits next to* **MARINA**.*)*

VANYA. It's a hundred degrees out and our renowned scholar is wearing a coat, gloves, galoshes, and carrying an umbrella.

ASTROV. The man looks out for himself.

VANYA. She's amazing, though, isn't she? Amazing! I've never seen a more beautiful woman in my life.

WAFFLES. *(To* **MARINA**.*)* Whenever I'm walking through fields, Marina, or strolling through the shady garden, or gazing at your wonderful table, I feel a kind of unfathomable bliss! The weather is enchanting, the birdies are singing, we're living here together in peace and harmony – what more do we need? *(Accepting a cup of tea.)* Tea! I'm so grateful.

VANYA. *(Dreamily.)* Her eyes... What an incredible woman!

ASTROV. Vanya!

VANYA. What?

ASTROV. What's new?

VANYA. Nothing. It's all old. I'm the same old me, maybe worse because I've gotten lazy. I don't do anything except sit around on my ass and complain like an old fart. And my mom, that feisty old crow, she's still just babbling non-stop about women's rights. She's got one foot in the grave, but she still believes a better world's a'comin'...

ASTROV. And the professor?

VANYA. Nothing! He just hides in his study all day writing, writing, crapping out boring essays nobody wants to read. I pity the paper! He'd be better off writing his autobiography – there's a gripping story! A retired academic, a rotting fish with a PhD. He has gout, rheumatism, migraines, his liver is swollen with jealousy and spite. And this poor rotting fish moves back into his late wife's house – no he's forced to move back here because he's too broke to live in the city, and he won't shut up about his bad luck, even though his luck is ridiculous! His dad was a church janitor, he got through school on scholarships, earned a bunch of fancy degrees, became a famous scholar, married two women who were way out of his league – fine, that's all kind of interesting. But get this: The man has been writing about art for twenty-five years, and he knows nothing about art! For twenty-five years he's been regurgitating other people's ideas about modernism, postmodernism, all that crap. For twenty-five years he's been writing about things smart people already know and stupid people don't care about. And with such self-regard! Such pretension! And now he's been "forced to retire" and nobody remembers his name. Which means that for twenty-five years he was just keeping some better man out of a job. But look at him – parading around like a demigod!

ASTROV. You sound jealous.

VANYA. Of course I'm jealous! Women love him! Don Juan couldn't hold a candle to this guy. My sister, a beautiful person – kind, generous, as pure as this blue sky – she gave him the best years of her life. And my mom – his *ex-mother-in-law* – she kisses the ground he walks on, to this day she follows him around like he's the Messiah. And his second wife, I mean, you saw her. She's gorgeous. Brilliant. And she married him when he was already an old man. Gave up her dreams for him. Why? For what?

ASTROV. Is she…faithful?

VANYA. Yes. Tragically.

ASTROV. Tragically? Why "tragically"?

VANYA. Because it doesn't mean anything. Cheat on an old man you can't stand – that's immoral. But stifle your true feelings and stay married to a man you don't love – that's moral?

WAFFLES. *(Fighting tears.)* Vanya, I hate it when you talk like this. You have to understand, the kind of person who would betray their wife or husband, that's a disloyal person. That's the kind of person who would betray their country!

VANYA. Turn off the fountain, Waffles!

WAFFLES. Hear me out, Vanya. My wife ran away with the man she loved the day after our wedding, thanks to my unappealing appearance. But I've never broken my vow. To this day, I love her and I'm faithful to her. I help her out whenever I can. I even gave her my house so that she would have a place to raise the babies she had with the man she loved. Sure, I gave up my happiness, but I still have my honor. And my wife? She's an old woman now, her beauty has succumbed to the laws of nature, and the man she loved has died. What does she have left?

*(***SONYA*** and ***YELENA*** enter. ***MARIA*** enters
with a book, sits down and begins to read.)*

SONYA. *(Anxious.)* Nanny, those men are back, will you
go talk to them? I'll take care of lunch.

*(***MARINA*** exits. ***SONYA*** pours tea. ***YELENA***
takes her cup and drinks, sitting on the
swing.)*

ASTROV. *(To* **YELENA**.*)* I took a look at your husband, like
you asked. I thought you said he was sick – rheumatism
and something else? Honestly, he seems fine. Maybe
healthier than the rest of us.

YELENA. Last night he was depressed and moaning about
the pain in his legs. But you're right, today he seems fine.

ASTROV. Yeah, well I almost killed myself rushing out
here. Never mind, it's not the first time. Maybe I'll stay
the night and at least get a little sleep.

SONYA. *(Delighted.)* Really? You never stay the night
anymore! I bet you haven't eaten, have you?

ASTROV. *(Playful.)* No ma'am, I haven't eaten.

SONYA. Then sit down. You have to join us for dinner, too.
We're eating late these days. *(She takes a drink of tea.)*
Ulch, this tea is cold!

WAFFLES. My apologies, the temperature in the teapot
has indeed plummeted.

YELENA. It's fine, we can drink it cold, Ivan.

WAFFLES. Excuse me, ma'am... my name's not Ivan, it's
Ilya, ma'am... Ilya Telegin, but most people call me
Waffles, on account of my pockmarked face. I'm Sonya's
godfather, and the professor, your spouse, knows me
quite well. I actually live here on your estate, ma'am.
You may have noticed that I eat dinner with you every
night.

SONYA. Ilya is our right hand man. Our rock. *(Tenderly, to* **WAFFLES.***)* Isn't that right, Godfather? Here let me pour you some more tea.

MARIA. Oh no!

SONYA. What is it Grandma?

MARIA. I forgot to tell Alexander something important – my memory is shot! *"Lethe, the river of oblivion rolls her watery labyrinth...!"* Anyway, I finally read the new essay by that friend of his...the one everybody's fighting about... Ha...

(Pause.)

ASTROV. Is it interesting?

MARIA. Oh it's interesting all right but it's also a piece of reactionary drivel. That crusty old dinosaur is attacking the same ideas he was marching for fifty years ago! It's shocking what's happening in this country!

VANYA. There's nothing shocking about it! Drink your tea, Mama.

MARIA. But it's important, we should be talking about it!

VANYA. We've been doing nothing but talking about this stuff for fifty years, Mom. Enough. None of it makes any difference.

MARIA. Why do you find the sound of my voice so unpleasant lately? Sweetheart, you've changed so much in the last year, I barely recognize you. What have you done with my son? I raised you to be a man of conviction! You were passionate and kind, you gave a damn about the world! My brilliant boy, my shining light...

VANYA. Oh yes! I was a shining light who shone on nothing and nobody... *(Beat.)* A shining light? Are you mocking me? Yes, I used to be just like you, Mom, blinding myself with *fake intellectualism* so I wouldn't have to see life for what it really is. I thought I was *doing something*.

But now – if you only knew! I can't sleep at night because I'm so angry, I'm so filled with rage at myself pissing away all that time when I was young and could have had everything I'm too old to have now!

SONYA. Uncle Vanya! Boring!

MARIA. You're blaming your former convictions but they're not guilty, sweetheart, you are! You forgot that without deeds, convictions mean nothing. They're dead letters. You should have *done something* –

VANYA. Done something – like what? We can't all be… *perpetual writing machines* like His Majesty Professor.

MARIA. What does that even mean?

SONYA. Grandma! Uncle Vanya! Please!

VANYA. I'll shut up. I'll shut up. I'm sorry.

(*Pause.*)

YELENA. Nice weather today… Not too hot.

(*Pause.*)

VANYA. Nice weather for hanging yourself.

(**WAFFLES** *tunes the guitar.*)

(**MARINA** *walks around the house calling the chickens.*)

MARINA. Cheep, cheep, cheep.

SONYA. What did they want, Nanny?

MARINA. Same old thing. I said we might have more work in the fall. (*Looking around.*) Cheep, cheep, cheep.

SONYA. Which one are you looking for?

MARINA. That speckled mama hen ran off with her babies again… I don't want the crows to eat them.

(She exits. Everyone listens silently as **WAFFLES** *plays a polka.* A **NEIGHBOR** *kid appears.)*

NEIGHBOR. Doctor? *(To* **ASTROV.***)* Sorry to bug you but the folks down at the orchard said they need you to come right away.

ASTROV. Oh yeah? Why?

NEIGHBOR. There's been some kind of accident.

MARIA. Ohhh…

ASTROV. *(Irritated.)* Thank you. Welp. Gotta go. *(Looks around for his hat.)* Damn, that's too bad.

SONYA. I'm so sorry. Come back for dinner when you're done.

ASTROV. Nah, it'll be too late. *(Re: his hat.)* What the hell… where did it go?

*(**MARINA** re-enters.)*

You know what, Marina? I'll have that shot of vodka now if you don't mind.

MARINA. Sure sweetie.

*(**MARINA** exits.)*

SONYA. *(To* **NEIGHBOR** *kid.)* Sit and eat something.

ASTROV. What the… where'd it go? *(He finds his hat.)* Remember that show about a man with a giant mustache and a tiny brain…? I am that man. *(To* **YELENA.***)* If you wanna come visit sometime – you and Sonya – I'd love that. My place is small, around seventy-five acres, but there's a first-rate orchard and a nursery, the only one

---

* A license to produce *Uncle Vanya* does not include a performance license for any third-party or copyrighted music. Licensees should create an original composition or use music in the public domain. For further information, please see the Music and Third-Party Materials Use Note on page iii.

of its kind for a hundred miles. And the state forest is right next door – the ranger's getting old, so I'm...ah... I'm taking care of the land.

YELENA. Oh I've heard all about your passion for saving the forests. I'm sure you do a lot of good but doesn't it interfere with your true calling? I mean...doctoring...

ASTROV. God only knows what our true calling is.

(YELENA *smiles.*)

YELENA. Is it interesting?

ASTROV. Yeah. The work is very interesting.

VANYA. Wildly!

YELENA. But you're so young, you look, what...thirty-six, thirty-seven? It can't be *that* interesting. Trees and more trees. God, that sounds monotonous.

SONYA. No, it's fascinating! The doctor plants a new forest every year – he's won all kinds of awards for it! And he's working to save the older forests too. He says that trees are the jewels of the earth, they teach us to understand beauty and inspire our higher feelings. Forests transform entire climate systems, they make them gentler and milder, and when humans don't have to fight so hard to survive...well then we can become gentler too. Kinder and more sensitive. Generous. More beautiful even. In gentler climates people become more optimistic, their speech is graceful, their attitudes toward women more enlightened and less hateful –

VANYA. Bravo, bravo, that's a very moving speech! (*To* ASTROV.) Makes me want to chop up a little wood for my fireplace.

ASTROV. Go ahead! You know I don't care about that. What I don't understand is why we're still cutting down billions of trees every year, when we know the homes of animals and birds are being demolished –

VANYA. Here we go!

ASTROV. – rivers are drying up, astonishing landscapes are disappearing from memory, all because we're too lazy and cynical to do anything to stop it! *(To* **YELENA.***)* Don't you agree? You'd have to be a monster to burn up all this beauty, to destroy what you cannot create. Humans are born with the intelligence and imagination to care for everything that's been given to us – but, no, we're obsessed with destruction. Every day, there are fewer and fewer forests, rivers are receding, we're wiping out whole branches from the tree of life –

(To **VANYA.***)* Don't give me that look! You think I'm naive...fine, maybe I am. But when I walk through a forest that I saved from being cut down, or I hear the wind rustling through the leaves of young trees, saplings I planted with my own hands, I feel like I have a tiny bit of power over the climate. When I plant a birch tree and watch it grow up, turn green, and sway in the wind... *(Noticing* **MARINA** *with the vodka.)* Never mind. I'm out of time. *(To* **MARINA.***)* Thank you.

> *(He takes the shot and downs it.)*

I'm a freak. I should hit the road. Thank you all for the wonderful company.

> *(He exits toward the house.* **SONYA** *takes his arm.)*

SONYA. When will you be back?

ASTROV. I don't know.

SONYA. *(As they exit.)* Don't make us wait a whole month again.

> *(***MARIA** *and* **WAFFLES** *remain at the table.* **YELENA** *and* **VANYA** *make their way to the porch.)*

YELENA. Why are you acting like this?

VANYA. What?

YELENA. You're behaving like a child! Why are you being so mean to your mother? And you picked a fight with Alexander again this morning. It's so petty!

VANYA. I know but I hate him.

YELENA. You have no reason to hate him, he's no worse than anybody else. Especially you.

VANYA. I wish you could see your face right now, the way you move. It's like you're too bored to live your life...

YELENA. Yes, I'm bored! You criticize my husband all day and every one of you looks at me as if you feel sorry for me: Poor thing, she married an old man! All of this sympathy for me – I know what you're doing! It's just like the doctor said: You're destroying the forests – pretty soon there will be nothing left –

VANYA. Wait, who's destroying the –?

YELENA. Men! You destroy the forests and you destroy other people the same way. Pretty soon there won't be any kindness or generosity or humanity left on the planet. Why can't you all just relax around a woman who doesn't belong to you? The doctor's right, there's a little demon of destruction inside every one of you. You have no respect for the forests, or for the birds, or for women, or for one another.

VANYA. I'm not loving this theory.

(Beat.)

YELENA. That doctor has such a tired, anxious face – what an interesting face. Sonya likes him, obviously. She's in love with him. I don't blame her. He's been out to visit three times since we got here. I haven't said a nice word to him, I'm too shy. I am! He probably thinks I'm a bitch. You know why you and I are such good friends, Vanya? Because we're both such boring, tedious people. Tedious! Don't look at me like that. I don't like it.

VANYA. How am I supposed to look at you? I love you. You're everything to me, you know that. I know the chances of you loving me back are small – zero – but I don't care. I don't need anything from you, Lena. Please just let me look at you. Let me listen to your voice.

YELENA. Shhhh. Your mother is right there.

(She goes toward the house. **VANYA** *follows her.)*

VANYA. Just let me talk about my love. That's all I need. That's enough to make me happy.

YELENA. This is torture.

(They both go into the house. **WAFFLES** *strikes the strings and plays a too-cheerful number.*[*] **MARIA** *writes something down in the margins of her article. Maybe she sings or hums along...)*

End of Act One

---

[*] A license to produce *Uncle Vanya* does not include a performance license for any third-party or copyrighted music. Licensees should create an original composition or use music in the public domain. For further information, please see the Music and Third-Party Materials Use Note on page iii.

ACT TWO

*(Night. The dining room. The **PROFESSOR** dozes in a chair. **YELENA** sits nearby.)*

PROFESSOR. *(Waking up.)* Who's that? Sonya is that you?

YELENA. It's me.

PROFESSOR. Oh sweet Lena... this pain is unbearable!

YELENA. Your blanket fell.

(She picks it up and lays it over his knees.)

I'll close the window.

PROFESSOR. No, it's suffocating in here. I dozed off and had a dream that my left leg belonged to someone else. The pain woke me up. It's *excruciating.* I'm sorry I don't care what they say, this isn't gout, it's rheumatism! What time is it now?

YELENA. Almost one.

(Pause.)

PROFESSOR. In the morning, look in the library and see if we have any Byron. I think he's in there.

YELENA. What...? Who's in there?

PROFESSOR. Find me some poems by Byron in the morning. I know we have some. Why is it so hard for me to breathe?

YELENA. You're tired. You haven't slept for two nights.

PROFESSOR. They say Milton's gout killed him! I'm afraid that's what's going to happen to me. Old age is disgusting. Goddammit! I hate getting old, it's repulsive. I'm disgusting. You all must think I'm disgusting.

YELENA. You act like it's everybody else's fault you got old.

PROFESSOR. You think I'm disgusting.

*(**YELENA** moves away from him.)*

You're right. I'm not stupid, I understand. You're young, you're beautiful, you're healthy, you want to live. And I'm an old man, practically a corpse. Right? You think I don't understand? It's stupid that I'm still alive. But you wait, I'll set you all free soon. Don't you worry, I won't drag it out much longer.

YELENA. I'm exhausted. Jesus Christ, stop talking.

PROFESSOR. Oh yes, thanks to me, everybody's exhausted, bored and has wasted the best years of their lives. I'm the only one who's happy and loving life!

YELENA. Shut up! You're torturing me!

PROFESSOR. Of course. I torture everyone. Apparently.

YELENA. *(Through tears.)* I can't take this! What do you want from me?

PROFESSOR. Nothing.

YELENA. Well then stop talking. Please.

PROFESSOR. It's weird, Vanya starts talking, or even Mama, that old windbag, and it's fine, everybody pays attention. But I say one word and suddenly you're all miserable. Even my voice is disgusting. Fine, let's say I am egotistical. I am! I'm a tyrant. Don't I have the right to be a bit egotistical at my age? Haven't I earned that? I'm really asking you, Lena. Don't I have the right to a peaceful old age, to some thoughtfulness and attention from people?

YELENA. No one is disputing your rights.

> *(The sound of wind slamming the window shut.)*

The wind is picking up.

> *(She covers him with the blanket.)*

It's going to rain. No one is disputing your rights.

PROFESSOR. A man devotes his entire life to art, to literature, to the pursuit of knowledge. He loves his cozy office, the thrill of the lecture hall, the company of his brilliant colleagues – and then suddenly, out of the blue, he finds himself living in this crypt. Surrounded by stupid people having stupid conversations. *(Beat.)* I want to live. I love success. I love being famous. I love the parties and the people and the noise and here – I'm in exile! I spend every minute dreaming about the past, reading about other people's successes, fearing death… I can't do it! I'm not strong enough! And not one of you will forgive me for getting old!

YELENA. Be patient. In five or six years, I'll be old too.

> *(**SONYA** enters.)*

SONYA. Dad, you made us send for the doctor and now you won't even talk to him? It's rude. We made him come all this way for no reason.

PROFESSOR. What do I need your doctor for? He knows as much about medicine as I know about astronomy.

SONYA. We can't call in a whole team of specialists to treat your gout.

PROFESSOR. I'm not talking to that lunatic!

SONYA. Do what you want. I don't care.

PROFESSOR. What time is it now?

YELENA. Almost one.

PROFESSOR. I feel like I'm suffocating. Sonya, give me my drops, they're on the table.

SONYA. Here.

(She hands him the drops.)

PROFESSOR. *(Irritated.)* No, not these! I can't ask you for anything!

SONYA. Stop being a baby. Maybe some people like it, but I don't have time for it. I have to get up early and deal with the hay.

*(Enter **VANYA** in his robe, carrying a light. He's a little drunk.)*

VANYA. There's a big storm a-comin'!

(Lightning.)

And there it is! Lena, Sonya. Go to bed, I'm here to take over.

PROFESSOR. No, no! Don't leave me with him! Please! He'll talk me to death!

VANYA. You have to let them rest! They haven't slept for two nights.

PROFESSOR. They can go to bed but you have to leave too! Please. I'm begging you. In the name of our former friendship. Go to bed. We'll talk later.

VANYA. *(With a grin.)* Our former friendship...

SONYA. Be quiet, Uncle Vanya.

PROFESSOR. *(To **SONYA**.)* Sweetheart, please don't leave me alone with him! He'll talk me to death!

VANYA. This is getting funny.

*(Enter **MARINA** with a light.)*

SONYA. You should go to bed, Nanny. It's late.

MARINA. Nobody cleared the table. How am I supposed to sleep?

(She walks to the **PROFESSOR.***)*

PROFESSOR. No one can sleep, everyone is suffering, I alone am happy.

MARINA. *(Tenderly.)* What is it, sweetie? Are you in pain? My legs hurt too, they're throbbing – dear God they hurt!

(She fixes the blanket.)

You've been in pain for such a long time, haven't you sweetie? Sonya's mama, God bless her soul, she could never sleep, either. She was always too worried about you... Sweet Faith, God bless her soul, she loved you so much.

*(***MARINA*** helps him up.)*

Old folks are like babies, they need people to feel sorry for them. But nobody feels sorry for old folks!

(She kisses him.)

Let's go, sweetie. To your comfy bed! Let's go, my little sunshine. I'll make you some tea and warm up your feet and pray for your pain to go away.

PROFESSOR. *(Touched.)* Let's go, Marina.

MARINA. My legs ache too! They throb! Throb, throb, throb! It's terrible.

(She leads him out. **SONYA** *helps.)*

Sonya's mama was always crying over you, poor thing. You were too young and silly to understand, Sonya. *(To* **PROFESSOR.***)* Let's get you to bed, sweetie, let's go... let's go.

*(***PROFESSOR***,* **SONYA***, and* **MARINA** *exit.)*

YELENA. He's killing me. I can barely stand up.

VANYA. He's killing you, and I'm killing myself. I haven't slept for three nights.

YELENA. Something's wrong in this house. Your mom hates everything, except politics and fawning over my husband. Alexander's irritated all the time, he doesn't trust me, he's afraid of you. Sonya's mad at her father, she's mad at me, she hasn't spoken to me in two weeks. You hate my husband and you're mean to your mother. I can't take it! I almost burst into tears twenty times today. It's this house, I'm telling you, things are not right in this house.

VANYA. No more theories, please!

YELENA. Vanya, you're a smart man. You know that the world is dying not just because of violence or wars or wildfires, but from all this hatred and hostility, from all of these petty little squabbles. You need to stop complaining about everyone and try to make peace, try to bring us all together.

VANYA. Help me make peace with myself first. *(Grabbing her hand.)* Lena...

YELENA. No. *(Pulling away.)* Get away.

VANYA. The rain will stop soon and everything in nature will breathe freely. Except me. I'm suffocating. Day and night, I can only think about one thing: that my life is gone and I will never get it back. I have no past, I wasted it on stupid things. And the present is painfully absurd. Here's my life, Lena. Here's my love. Where do I put it? What do I do with it? My love is dying, it's like a ray of sunlight disappearing into a pit, and I'm dying too.

YELENA. When you talk to me about love, my mind goes blank and I don't know what to say. I'm sorry, there's nothing I can say to you. Good night.

VANYA. Lena, it kills me that there's another life wasting away in this house, right next to mine! Yours! Your life! What are you waiting for? What is keeping you here?

YELENA. Vanya! You're drunk!

VANYA. Possibly. Possibly.

YELENA. Where's the doctor?

VANYA. He's in bed...in my room. I'm possibly drunk. Anything is possible!

YELENA. Why did you get drunk again?

VANYA. So I can pretend I'm alive. Don't judge me, Lena.

YELENA. You never used to drink like this and you talked a lot less too. Go to bed. I'm tired of you.

VANYA. *(Grabbing her hand.)* Oh Lena...you're amazing!

YELENA. Jesus, leave me alone. This is repulsive.

(She's gone.)

VANYA. She's gone.

(Beat.)

I met her at my sister's house ten years ago. Why didn't I fall in love with her then? We'd be married now. Yes... the storm would wake us up, she'd be scared of the thunder, and I would hold her in my arms: "Don't be scared. I'm here." Oh God, I'm all mixed up. Why am I old? Why doesn't she understand me? I can't stand her self-righteousness, her stupid theories about the "dying world" – God I hate them.

(Pause.)

I was conned! I worshiped the professor, I did. I loved him. I worked like a dog for him. Woke up at five every morning. Never took a day off. Squeezed every last drop out of this farm and sent him everything we made to support his work because I thought he was some kind of genius! Oh my God, and now? He's old and not one page of his work will survive him. He's a nothing! A failure! He conned me... I was conned...

(**ASTROV** *enters in his suit coat, without shirt or tie. He's drunk.* **WAFFLES** *follows with a guitar.*)

ASTROV. Play something!

WAFFLES. Everybody's sleeping.

ASTROV. Plaaaaaaaaaay!

(**WAFFLES** *plays softly.*)

(*To* **VANYA**.) You alone? No ladies?

(*Arms wide,* **ASTROV** *sings softly.*)

IT WAS ON THE GOOD SHIP VENUS
BY CHRIST, YA SHOULD'VE SEEN US
THE FIGUREHEAD WAS A GIRL IN BED
AND THE MAST AN ENORMOUS –

Whoa. Some rainstorm. What time is it?

VANYA. How the hell should I know?

ASTROV. Did I hear Yelena out here?

VANYA. She left.

ASTROV. God what a *sumptuous* woman...

(*He studies the bottles on the table.*)

Whoa. Lotta medicine. Wow. Prescriptions from three different cities – he's annoying the whole country with his gout! Is he really sick or is he pretending?

VANYA. Oh, he's sick.

(*Pause.*)

ASTROV. Why are you so sad? You feel sorry for the professor?

VANYA. Leave me alone.

ASTROV. Or maybe you're in love with Mrs. Professor?

VANYA. She's my friend.

ASTROV. Already?

VANYA. What do you mean "already"?

ASTROV. Women and men can only become friends in this order: First acquaintances, then lovers, and, only then, friends.

VANYA. That's vulgar.

ASTROV. Really? Yeah, I know. I'm becoming *vulgar*. I'm also wasted in case you can't tell. I get drunk like this about once a month now and whoooo, when I'm in this condition, I get so cocky, there's no stopping me! I take on the most complicated surgeries and perform them *brilliantly*. I make sweeping plans for the future of humanity...and I don't feel like a freak! I know that my talents are of massive importance to humankind! Massive! I'm a God at the center of my own perfect philosophical system, and all of you, my dear brothers, are just...tiny little bugs. Microbes. *(To* **WAFFLES**.*)* Waffles! Play!

WAFFLES. My wonderful friend, I'd love to with all my heart, but you have to understand the whole house is sleeping!

ASTROV. Play!

(**WAFFLES** *strums very softly.)*

We should probably drink a little more. I think there's some cognac somewhere. And when the sun comes up we can move the party to my place! Lezzzgooo! I've got this assistant who never says "let's go" he always says "lezzzgooo!" He's a total crook. So – lezzzgooo?

ASTROV. *(Seeing* **SONYA** *enter.)* Excuse me, I've got no shirt on.

(He exits quickly. **WAFFLES** *follows.)*

SONYA. Uncle Vanya, you got drunk with the doctor again? He's always like this, but you? You're too old for this. It's embarrassing.

VANYA. What is age? Besides, when you've got no life, you have to live in a mirage. Eh. It's better than nothing.

SONYA. The hay's going to rot if we don't get it moved and you're living in a mirage! You've given up running this place! I'm doing everything by myself. I can't take it. I'm exhausted. *(Startled.)* Are you crying?

VANYA. What? No. I'm fine... it's silly. The way you looked at me just now... your mother used to look at me like that. Oh God. *(Kissing her hands and face desperately.)* My sister, my beautiful sister. *(Beat.)* Where is she now? If she only knew! If she only knew!

SONYA. What? Knew what?

VANYA. Nothing. It's too horrible... I'll go now.

(He leaves. After a beat, the sound of someone in the darkness.)

SONYA. Doctor! Is that you? Can we talk?

ASTROV. *(From the darkness.)* Coming.

(He appears.)

How may I help you, *ma'am*?

SONYA. Go ahead and drink yourself stupid if it means that much to you, but don't get my uncle drunk. It's bad for him.

ASTROV. *(Playful.)* Yes, ma'am! We won't drink anymore. I should go home. Sun'll be up soon.

SONYA. What? No! It's raining. Wait till morning.

ASTROV. I'll be fine. Just please, don't make me talk to your father again. I tell him it's gout, he says it's rheumatism. I ask him to lie down, he sits up. And today, he wouldn't speak to me at all.

SONYA. He's spoiled. *(Looking around.)* Would you like a snack?

ASTROV. ...Yeah. Why not?

SONYA. I love a little snack in the middle of the night. *(Rifling around for food.)* People say my father had too much success with women and it spoiled him. Here, have some cheese.

(They stand and eat together.)

ASTROV. Haven't eaten a thing all day, I just drank. Your dad's a difficult man. *(Picks up a bottle of something.)* May I? *(Takes a swig.)* Since we're alone, can I be honest with you...? I wouldn't last a month in this house. I'd die here. Your father doesn't give a crap about anything except his gout, your uncle whines non-stop, your grandma, well your grandma is her own special case. And your *stepmother*...

SONYA. What about my stepmother?

ASTROV. Everything about a person should be beautiful: their face, their soul, their mind. She's gorgeous, no question, but she doesn't do anything! She just eats, sleeps, and enchants all of us with her beauty. She's got no responsibilities. No work. It's a meaningless life, am I right?

(Pause.)

Maybe I'm being too hard on her. I'm unhappy with life just like your uncle, we're a couple of assholes.

SONYA. Are you really "unhappy with life"?

ASTROV. I mean I love life in theory. But this backwoods, stupid, philistine life – I hate it. And my own personal life, oh God, there's not one good thing about it. You know when you're walking through the forest on a dark night, and you see a little light shining in the distance and you suddenly stop thinking about how tired you are? You don't notice the darkness anymore, or the prickly branches scratching your face...? I work, you know this, I work harder than anyone in this county, but life just keeps beating me down – some days I don't know how I'm going to keep going – but there's no little light in the distance for me. I don't hope for anything anymore. I don't love anybody... I haven't loved anybody for a long time.

SONYA. Nobody?

ASTROV. Nobody. I mean, I feel a kind of tenderness for your nanny, but that's just nostalgia. The people out here are crude and ignorant, but honestly the "educated" ones are even worse. They're so petty, they have no concept of what life is like outside their little bubble. They're neurotic, self-obsessed, hysterical. They meet someone new, they're suspicious. "He must be a psychopath!" And when they're not sure what label to paste on *my* forehead, they call me weird. I'm a weird, weird man. I love the forest – that's weird. I don't eat meat – weird. It's like we can't have any kind of authentic connection with nature anymore, or with one another. Nope!

(He reaches for a drink. She stops him.)

SONYA. Please don't drink anymore.

ASTROV. Why not?

SONYA. It's not who you are! You're sensitive, kind, you have such a gentle voice. You're not like other people – you're beautiful. Why would you want to get drunk all the time and throw your life away like everybody else? Please, don't do it! You keep saying we destroy everything that's been given to us, so why would you destroy yourself? Don't do it, please. I'm begging you. Please, don't do it. Please. Don't drink anymore.

ASTROV. *(Offering her his hand.)* Done. I will not drink anymore.

SONYA. Give me your word.

ASTROV. You have my word.

SONYA. Thank you.

ASTROV. Ta-da, I'm sober! See? Now I'm totally sober and I'll stay this way until I die. *(Looks at his watch.)* Where were we? Oh yeah: My time has passed, I'm old, I'm overworked, my feelings have all gone numb, I don't love anybody...and I never will. The only thing that still excites me is beauty. Beauty still gets to me. I think if your stepmother wanted to, she could make me lose my mind. But that's not love... that's not real...

(He closes his eyes for a moment.)

SONYA. What's wrong?

ASTROV. I... ah. I lost that patient a few months ago, right after I put him under.

SONYA. It's time for you to forget about that.

(Pause.)

Doctor...? If I had a friend, or a younger sister, and I told you that she... well what if I told you she was in love with you, how do you think you would respond?

ASTROV. I don't know. I probably wouldn't respond. I'd try to make her understand that I'm not capable of loving her back. *(Beat.)* Anyway. I should go if I'm ever going to get out of here. Let's say goodbye, sweetheart, or we'll keep talking till morning. I'll sneak out this way so your uncle doesn't try to stop me.

*(**ASTROV** exits. **SONYA** is left alone.)*

SONYA. He didn't say anything really. His heart is still a complete mystery. So why do I feel so happy? *(Laughing.)* I said: You're sensitive, beautiful, you have such a gentle voice – was that ridiculous? I can still hear his voice whispering in my ears, it's like I can feel him in the air... When I said that thing about a younger sister, he didn't get it. *(Pacing.)* Oh I hate that I'm not beautiful! And I know I'm not beautiful, I know it. When I was leaving church on Sunday I heard some women talking about me: "She's so hard-working, what a nice girl. Too bad she didn't get her mother's looks..."

*(**YELENA** enters.)*

YELENA. *(Opening the windows.)* The storm has passed. The air feels so good!

(Pause.)

Where's the doctor?

SONYA. He left.

YELENA. Sonya!

SONYA. What?

YELENA. How long are you going to stay mad at me? Neither of us has done anything wrong. Why do we have to be enemies? I'm tired of it.

SONYA. I know... I know. I've been wanting to make up... *(She embraces her.)* I'm sorry. I'm not angry anymore.

YELENA. Finally. Thank God.

(They are both moved.)

SONYA. Is Dad asleep?

YELENA. No, he's just sitting in the living room. *(Beat.)* You and I haven't spoken for weeks, Sonya, it doesn't make any sense...

(**YELENA** *sees the leftovers.*)

Oooh what is this...?

SONYA. The doctor had a snack.

YELENA. Oh yeah? Ha. And there's wine... let's drink to our friendship!

SONYA. Yes, please, let's have a toast.

YELENA. Here we'll drink from the same glass to make it official... *(Pouring.)* Like this.

(**YELENA** *wraps her right arm around* **SONYA**'s *so that they can drink with their arms entwined.*)

So... To friendship?

SONYA. To friendship!

(They take a drink and embrace.)

I've been wanting to make up for such a long time but I felt so ashamed, I'm not sure why... *(She starts to cry.)*

YELENA. Why are you crying?

SONYA. I don't know. I just am.

YELENA. Oh sweetie. It's all right, you're all right... *(Starts to cry.)* You weirdo, now I'm crying too...

(Pause.)

You think I married your father because he was famous. But I swear to you on my life – whatever that means – I married him for love. I was crazy about him, everybody was! He was brilliant and charismatic and *alive*, and when a man like that shines his light on you… *(Beat.)* It wasn't real love, I know that now, but it seemed real to me at the time. Please don't judge me. Sonya. Ever since our wedding, whenever you look at me with those intelligent, suspicious eyes, it's like you're trying to kill me.

SONYA. I know, I know. I'm so sorry! I'm not mad anymore, I'm not! Truce! Let's put it all behind us, please.

YELENA. You shouldn't look at people that way, it doesn't suit you. We have to trust one another, don't you think, otherwise how are we supposed to get through life?

(Pause.)

SONYA. Tell me, as a friend… Are you happy?

YELENA. No.

SONYA. I knew it! One more question. Tell me, honestly – as a friend – do you wish you had a younger husband?

YELENA. You're such a little girl. Of course I do! *(Laughing.)* Ask me something else. Go ahead, ask me anything…

SONYA. Do you like the doctor?

YELENA. Yes, very much.

*(***SONYA*** laughs.)*

SONYA. I look so stupid right now, don't I? He's gone but I can still hear his voice in the air and when I close my eyes, all I see is his face – no please let me finish, I have to tell you something. *(Beat.)* No, never mind, it's too embarrassing. Let's go to my room, so we can talk in private. Do you think I'm an idiot? Be honest…! Will you talk to me about him? Tell me something. Tell me anything…

YELENA. Like what?

SONYA. He's so smart! He knows everything, he can do everything. He plants trees, he heals people...

YELENA. Oh sweetie. It's not about the trees, that man has *talent*. Do you know what talent is? It's having vision, imagination, a kind of free and restless mind. When he plants a little tree, he's dreaming about what it will become in a hundred years, he's creating the future. People like that are rare, we have to love them. *(Beat.)* Sure he drinks, he's rude sometimes – so what? A man like that can't be a saint. Think about what his life is like! Traveling day and night to take care of mean, stupid people, dealing with poverty and sickness and death. You can't expect a man like that to make it to forty sober!

*(**YELENA** kisses **SONYA**.)*

You deserve happiness, Sonya, you do. I want you to be happy with all my heart. Me? I'm boring. A minor character... In music, in my husband's life, in all of my romances... I've always been a minor character. You know what, sweetheart, now that I'm thinking about it, I am actually very, very unhappy! *(Pacing.)* I don't know if I'll ever be happy. Maybe I won't – why are you laughing?

SONYA. I'm sorry. I'm just so happy. I'm so happy.

YELENA. I want to play the piano. Yes! I feel like playing something...

SONYA. Oh yes I want you to play! *(Hugging her.)* I can't sleep. Play something!

YELENA. Yes! I'm going to play piano. I'm going to play something right now! Wait, your dad's still awake. When he's in one of his moods, music drives him crazy. Go ask him if he minds. If it won't bother him, I'll play. Go ask him.

SONYA. I'll be right back!

(**SONYA** *exits.*)

(**YELENA** *is alone for some time.*)

(**SONYA** *comes back.*)

SONYA. He said no.

End of Act Two

ACT THREE

(Daytime. The living room of the house. **VANYA** *and* **SONYA** *sit.* **YELENA** *paces.)*

VANYA. His Majesty the Professor has made his wishes known: We are to assemble here – in the living room – at one o'clock sharp. He has an important proclamation to make.

(He looks at his watch.)

Quarter to one. The suspense is killing me.

YELENA. He probably just wants to talk about the business.

VANYA. What does he know about the business? He doesn't do anything except write a bunch of bullshit, complain non-stop, and eat himself alive with jealousy –

SONYA. Uncle Vanya!

VANYA. I know, I know.

(He points at **YELENA**.*)*

Look at her. She's so bored, she's just staggering around. It's adorable.

YELENA. Buzz, buzz, buzz, you're like a little fly. Aren't you sick of your own voice? *(In agony.)* God I really am dying of boredom, I don't know what to do with myself.

SONYA. There's so much to do!

YELENA. Like what?

SONYA. You could help with the farm, or get a job teaching. You could go into town and volunteer at a shelter. There's so much to do! Before you and Dad came, Uncle Vanya and I sold produce at the market every week –

YELENA. I don't know how to do any of that! Besides, it's not interesting. Volunteer at a shelter? That's like the plot of some terrible novel. And what, I'm supposed to wake up one day and suddenly know how to be a teacher?

SONYA. You'd figure it out if you gave it a chance. *(Hugging her.)* Don't be bored, sweetheart. It's contagious. *(Laughing.)* Look at Uncle Vanya, he's stopped doing anything, he just follows you around like a shadow. The second you show up, I drop all my chores and come running to talk to you. And the doctor! He used to visit once a month if we were lucky – now he's here every day. He's forgotten all about his patients and his forests. You're some kind of sorceress.

VANYA. Why are you wasting away out here? *(Enthusiastic.)* Get out of here while you still can! You have mermaid blood flowing through your veins – so be a mermaid! Let yourself go for once in your life, fall head over heels in love with some water spirit, and dive into the ocean – leave me and your husband and all the rest of us poor sad men standing on the shore...

YELENA. Stop it – that's so mean.

VANYA. I'm sorry. I'm sorry. Forgive me.

(He kisses her hand.)

Truce.

YELENA. You're so annoying and you know it.

VANYA. I'm going to bring you a bouquet of roses, as a peace offering. I cut a beautiful bunch for you this morning. Autumn roses – sad and lovely...

(He exits.)

SONYA. "Autumn roses – sad and lovely..."

(They look out the window.)

YELENA. September already. How are we going to make it through the winter?

(Pause.)

Where's the doctor?

SONYA. In Uncle Vanya's room. I need to talk to you.

YELENA. About what?

SONYA. About *what*?

*(She snuggles up to **YELENA**.)*

YELENA. Oh sweetheart. *(Petting her hair.)* It will be all right. It will. I promise.

SONYA. I'm not beautiful.

YELENA. You have such pretty hair.

SONYA. No! When a woman isn't beautiful, people always say "You have such pretty eyes, you have such pretty hair..." I've loved him for six years! I love him more than my own mother. Even when he's not around, I can hear the sound of his voice, I can feel the touch of his hands. I've spent years staring at that door, just waiting for him to walk through, and now he comes here every day but he never even looks at me. He doesn't see me. *(Hopeless.)* Oh God, help me please. I've been praying but it doesn't help. The second he shows up, I run to him and start babbling. I've lost all my pride, I can't control myself. Yesterday, I couldn't help it, I told Uncle Vanya everything. He knows I'm in love, you all know. Everybody knows.

YELENA. Does he know?

SONYA. No. He doesn't see me.

YELENA. He's a weird man. *(Beat.)* You know what? Let me talk to him. I'll be discreet... I'll just hint.

(Pause.)

How much longer can you go on without knowing the truth? Let me talk to him!

*(**SONYA** nods.)*

Good. He loves you or he doesn't – let's find out. Don't be embarrassed, sweetheart, I'll be subtle about it, he won't even know it's happening. We just need to find out: Yes, or no.

(Pause.)

And if it's no, he should stop coming here. Yes?

*(A beat. **SONYA** nods.)*

It will be easier if you don't have to see him. We can't stick our heads in the sand forever, let's find out. He promised to show me some of his paintings. Go tell him I'd love to see them right now.

SONYA. *(Excited.)* You'll tell me the truth!

YELENA. Of course. I think the truth – whatever it might be – is never as bad as not knowing. You can trust me.

SONYA. Yes...okay. I'll tell him you want to see his paintings...

(She stops by the door.)

No, I can't... not knowing is better. At least then there's still hope.

YELENA. What are you talking about?

SONYA. Nothing.

*(**SONYA** leaves.)*

YELENA. There's nothing worse than knowing someone's secret and not being able to help. He's not in love with her, that's clear, but why shouldn't he marry her? She'd make a wonderful wife for a country doctor. She's smart, kind, loving...

(*Pause.*)

I know exactly how she feels, poor girl. Stuck out here in the middle of nowhere with a bunch of gray blobs who pass for people, watching them do nothing except eat, sleep, and drink – and then he walks in. He's beautiful, interesting, alive. Like a bright moon on a dark night. What would it be like to fall under his spell, to lose yourself, to forget about everything and everyone else? Oh no... maybe I'm a little bit under his spell too. I'm so bored when he's not here... (*Beat.*) Vanya says there's mermaid blood in my veins. "*Let yourself go for once in your life.*" Maybe I should. I'll fly away from all of you, free as a bird. I'll fly far away from your stupid conversations and forget that any of you ever existed. (*Beat.*) But no. My conscience won't let me... I'm a coward...

(**ASTROV** *enters.*)

ASTROV. Hello. (*Beat.*) You wanted to see my paintings?

YELENA. Yes. You promised to show me what you're working on. (*Beat.*) Are you free now?

ASTROV. Ah...yeah. Sure.

(*Pause. He begins to tack a map to the wall. She moves in to help him. After a bit.*)

What did you study in college?

YELENA. (*Helping him with the map.*) Music.

ASTROV. Ah.

YELENA. I went to a conservatory.

ASTROV. Oh, okay! Well this probably won't be very interesting for you, then.

YELENA. Why not? I'm interested in all kinds of things.

(**ASTROV** *continues setting up his maps.*)

ASTROV. I have my own little table in Vanya's room. When I get so tired I can't think anymore, I come here and lose myself in this project for a few hours. Vanya and Sonya pay bills and I sit next to them and paint. It's cozy and peaceful... I like the sounds of the crickets chirping. Of course, I don't allow myself that much fun all the time, maybe once a month...

(*He points to the map.*)

See here? This is a painting of what our county looked like a hundred years ago. The light green sections – and the darker greens here – these are all forests. More than half of this region was covered with trees. The red cross-hatching right here on top of the green, indicates that, ah, moose and deer and cottontails lived there... I'm showing both flora and fauna. Oh, and this lake! You had your swans, geese, ducks, a big ole mess o' birds. That's what the old-timers like to say. *"There were once so many birds in these parts, they looked like giant black clouds flying overhead... they could block out the sun for hours."* And beyond the forests, there were all these little farms, see? Churches, watermills. Lotta horses and cows. I've ah, chosen to represent those with the color blue. See how thick this paint is here? That represents a whole herd of horses. They say every house in town used to have three horses.

(*Pause.*)

Now let's take a look down here. This is how it looked fifty years ago. Now the forest only takes up a third of the map. And the moose are all gone, and the fallow deer, and the wild pigeons and the little brown bats.

You can see the green and blue paint is much lighter here. *(Beat.)* Let's move on to the third one. This is us right now – this is the present. The moose have made a small comeback, sure, but now the wood grouse have disappeared and the cottontails are nearly extinct and the porcupines and the butterflies and the piping plover – along with most of the old-growth forests. What we're looking at here is a picture of relentless destruction that just keeps speeding up, in ten maybe twenty years, total obliteration. Now I know what you're gonna say, this is how the world works, the old way of life dies to make way for the new. And maybe I'd agree with you if in place of these forests, we were building beautiful schools or clinics, if we were creating things that made people healthier or smarter or happier – but that's not what's happening out here. All of this is being destroyed without any plan for the future, without any thought of tomorrow. *(Coolly.)* You're not interested in this. I can tell by your face.

YELENA. Maybe I don't fully understand it...

ASTROV. It's pretty simple. You're just not interested.

YELENA. Honestly, I was thinking about something else. I'm sorry. I need to...conduct a little interrogation, and I'm embarrassed. I don't know how to start.

ASTROV. Interrogation?

YELENA. Yes but it's all very innocent, don't get anxious. Let's sit down.

> *(They sit.)*

It's about, well, it's about a certain person we both know. And we can talk honestly, right, as friends, no hidden agendas? We'll talk and then we can forget everything we talked about. All right?

ASTROV. All right.

YELENA. It's about my stepdaughter, Sonya. Do you like her?

ASTROV. Yes, I respect her.

YELENA. Do you like her as a woman?

ASTROV. *(Not right away.)* No.

YELENA. This is almost over, I promise. Have you...noticed anything?

ASTROV. No.

(She takes his hand.)

YELENA. You don't love her, I can tell. But she's in pain, you have to understand that and...well you have to stop coming here.

*(**ASTROV** stands up.)*

ASTROV. Yeah. My time's up for that kind of thing anyway. I should go. I've got... *(He shrugs.)* Work.

(He's embarrassed.)

YELENA. Ugh what a terrible conversation! I feel like I've been carrying a huge weight on my shoulders. Thank God it's over! Let's pretend we never talked about this and...and you'll leave, right? You're a smart man. You understand.

(Pause.)

My face is getting hot.

ASTROV. You know, if you'd told me this a month ago I might have thought about it, but now...? If she's in pain, yes, I should leave. But there's something I don't understand: Why did you have to *interrogate* me? *(He looks her in the eyes.)* You are so devious.

YELENA. What does that mean?

ASTROV. *(Laughing.)* You're devious! All right, Sonya is in pain, but why did you need to perform some big interrogation? You know why I come here every day.

You know who I come to see. Don't look at me like that, you charming predator, I'm not some innocent kid.

YELENA. *(Confused.)* Predator? What are you talking about?

ASTROV. You're like a beautiful fluffy little weasel – you need victims! Look at me, I haven't worked in a month, I quit everything so I can chase after you, and you love it *so much*. Fine, you've defeated me, you knew that before the interrogation. I surrender. Go ahead, rip me to pieces.

YELENA. You're out of your mind!

ASTROV. *(Laughing.)* Oh right, you're so shy.

YELENA. I'm a better person than you think I am!

ASTROV. Fine, I'll leave right now and I won't come back, but tell me please... *(Takes her hand.)* How can we see each other? Where should we meet? Tell me where. Hurry, someone might come in, just tell me where to meet you. *(Passionate.)* God you are dazzling. Look at you. Can I kiss you? Can I just kiss your hair? It smells incredible...

YELENA. Stop it. I swear to you –

ASTROV. Don't swear, don't say anything. You are so beautiful. Look at your hands.

(He kisses her hands. She doesn't pull away.)

YELENA. You have to go now. *(Not moving away.)* This is out of control.

ASTROV. Tell me where we can meet. This is inevitable, it's going to happen and you know it.

*(They kiss. **VANYA** enters with roses. They don't notice him.)*

YELENA. Please get out of here. You know I can't do this.

ASTROV. Come see me tomorrow afternoon. Yeah? Yes? Will you come?

(*YELENA sees **VANYA**. Embarrassed, she moves away from **ASTROV**.*)

YELENA. This is horrible.

(**VANYA** *drops the bouquet.*)

VANYA. Don't worry about it. It's nothing, it's nothing. Yeah. Don't worry about it.

ASTROV. *(Nonchalant.)* Weather's not too bad today, eh? Lotta clouds this morning – looked like it was going to rain, but now it's sunny. Gonna be a beautiful autumn... winter crops shouldn't be too bad this year either.

(**ASTROV** *rolls up his map.*)

I just wish the days weren't getting shorter...

(*He exits.* **YELENA** *turns to* **VANYA**.)

YELENA. You have to help me get out of this house today. My husband and I need to leave this place today. You hear me? Today.

VANYA. *(Wiping his face.)* Ah, yeah? Well, okay... I saw everything, Lena, everything...

YELENA. Did you hear me? I have to leave this house today.

(*Enter the* **PROFESSOR, WAFFLES, SONYA,** *and* **MARINA**.)

WAFFLES. I, myself, am not feeling at the top of my game either, Professor. I've been a bit wobbly the past few days. And my head is pounding and pounding –

PROFESSOR. Where is everybody? This house is some kind of labyrinth. Twenty-six rooms, people wander off and you never see them again!

(*He rings his little bell.*)

Someone please go find Mama and Yelena.

YELENA. I'm right here.

PROFESSOR. Ladies and gentlemen, please take your seats.

(**SONYA** *approaches* **YELENA** *impatiently.*)

SONYA. *(Re:* **ASTROV.***)* Well, what did he say?

YELENA. Later.

PROFESSOR. *(To* **WAFFLES.***)* A man can make peace with sickness, I agree. What I can't stomach is the bewildering pace of country life.

SONYA. Why are you shaking? Are you upset?

(Looking into her face with curiosity.)

PROFESSOR. It feels like I've fallen from Earth onto some alien planet.

SONYA. He...he said he's not coming back here again, didn't he?

PROFESSOR. Please take your seats, ladies and gentlemen.

SONYA. Tell me. He's not coming back?

(**YELENA** *nods.*)

PROFESSOR. Sonya.

(**SONYA***'s not listening.*)

Sonya!

(Pause.)

She can't hear me. Nanny, you sit down too.

(**MARINA** *sits.*)

Friends, Romans, Countrymen!

VANYA. *(Agitated.)* Am I really needed here? Can I go?

PROFESSOR. No, Vanya. We need you most of all.

VANYA. How may I be of service, Your Majesty?

PROFESSOR. Why are you so angry?

> *(Pause.)*

If I've done you any wrong or...hurt your feelings in some way, please forgive me.

VANYA. Oh stop it. Let's get down to business. What do you need?

> *(**MARIA** enters.)*

PROFESSOR. And here she is, everybody, our beloved Mama!

> *(**MARIA** appreciates this fanfare.)*

MARIA. A community meeting – how wonderful!

PROFESSOR. Now that Mama is here, we can finally begin.

MARIA. What's on the agenda?

PROFESSOR. My friends, I've gathered you here today to announce that...an Inspector-General is coming! No, in all seriousness, I'm here to ask for your help and advice and, knowing your generosity, I hope to receive both. I'm a humble scholar, a bookish man, and I've always been a bit baffled by practical matters. I would never have survived all these years without the guidance of practical people like yourselves. And so I'm asking you Vanya, and you too Ilya, and of course, you darling Mama...

> *(Pause.)*

The fact is: *manet omnes una ox.* That is, *the same night awaits us all.* I'm getting older and the time has come for me to put my affairs in order for the sake of my family. I'm not thinking of myself, of course, I've lived a very full life. But I do have a younger wife and an unmarried daughter.

(Beat.)

It's impossible for me to keep living out here. We're just not country people! And we can't afford to live in the city on the income we make from this farm. We could, perhaps, sell off the woodlands, but that would be a one-shot deal and we need something that guarantees a regular yearly income. I have come up with one possible solution and I'd love to present it to you for discussion. Skipping the details, here's the big picture: Our estate yields, on average, no more than two percent annually. I propose we sell it. If we invest the money in stocks and bonds, we would increase our earnings to four, maybe five percent, and even generate a nice surplus we could use to buy a little cottage by the beach –

VANYA. Wait, what? I don't think I heard that right. Repeat what you just said.

PROFESSOR. We invest the money in stocks and bonds, and use the surplus to buy a little beach house.

VANYA. No, no not the beach house! You said something before that.

PROFESSOR. I propose we sell the estate.

VANYA. Yes, that's it. You'll sell the estate, excellent, what a great idea. *(Beat.)* And where do you think I should go with my poor old mother and Sonya here?

PROFESSOR. We can discuss all of that. We don't have to figure everything out right now.

VANYA. Hold on. I guess I don't understand how the world works, because I was stupid enough to think this estate belonged to Sonya. My late father bought this farm for my sister. And maybe I'm naive – maybe I'm thinking of thirteenth-century feudal law or something – it was my understanding that this estate passed from my sister to her daughter Sonya.

PROFESSOR. Yes of course it belongs to Sonya! Who's arguing with you? I would never sell the farm without Sonya's consent. Besides, I would be selling it for Sonya's benefit.

VANYA. This is insane, it's insane! Either I'm going crazy or – or –

MARIA. Sweetheart, calm down. We're having a civilized discussion. You need to hear what Alexander has to say.

VANYA. Give me some water. *(Drinks.)* Keep talking, keep talking. Say whatever you want.

PROFESSOR. I don't understand why you're so upset. I'm not saying my proposal is perfect. If everyone thinks it's a bad idea, I won't insist.

(Pause.)

WAFFLES. *(Embarrassed.)* I have a great respect for scholarship, sir – Professor. Actually more than respect, I have a family connection: My brother's wife's brother, his name is Gregory, maybe you've run into him at the university, he got his master's degree in –

VANYA. Waffles, no! We're talking business! *(To the* **PROFESSOR.***)* Wait – actually why don't you ask Waffles what he thinks? We bought the estate from his uncle.

PROFESSOR. Why do I need to ask him what he thinks?

VANYA. We bought this farm for two hundred thousand, way back when. My father paid seventy and there was a hundred thirty left on the mortgage. Now listen! My father would never have been able to afford that if I hadn't given up my own inheritance for the sake of my beautiful sister, because I loved her. And then, after giving up all my money, I worked like a dog for thirty years to pay off the rest of the mortgage –

PROFESSOR. I regret starting this conversation.

VANYA. The only reason this farm is free of debt is because of my personal efforts. And now that I'm old, you want to kick me out on my ass!

PROFESSOR. I don't understand what you want!

VANYA. I've been running this farm for twenty-five years, working my ass off for you, sending you money, and in all this time you have never once thanked me. All these years, I made barely enough to get by – and not once did you think to give me a raise! It never occurred to you to add even one penny to my salary!

PROFESSOR. But Vanya, how could I have known? I'm not a practical man. I don't understand these kinds of things. Why didn't you give yourself a raise? You could have done that any time you wanted!

VANYA. You mean, why didn't I steal? Oh now you all hate me because I didn't steal? Oh my God, I should have stolen – maybe now I wouldn't be fucking homeless!

MARIA. *(Sternly.)* Vanya.

WAFFLES. Vanya, my dear friend, don't do this. Don't destroy your own family. Don't do it.

VANYA. *(To the **PROFESSOR**.)* For twenty-five years, my mother and I have been trapped in this house, like little moles, and all we ever talked about was you. Your work, your life, your achievements. We were so proud of you, we spoke about you like you were some kind of god. We wasted all of our evenings talking about your books, and now I despise every word of them!

WAFFLES. Don't do this Vanya...

VANYA. We thought you were a genius, we quoted you, we memorized whole passages of your books. *(Beat.)* But now my eyes are finally open! I see everything! You write about art and you don't understand a goddamned thing about art! You were conning us!

PROFESSOR. Make him stop or I'm leaving!

YELENA. Vanya, I order you to shut up. Do you hear me?

VANYA. I will not shut up. *(Standing in the* **PROFESSOR**'s *way.)* Wait, I'm not finished! You destroyed my life! I didn't live, I didn't live! I sacrificed the best years of my life for you. You are my mortal enemy.

WAFFLES. I can't take this, I can't, I'm leaving...

(He exits, very upset.)

PROFESSOR. What do you want from me? And what right do you have to speak to me like this? You're a nothing! A nobody! If the farm is yours, take it, I don't need it!

YELENA. This is hell! I have to get out of here!

VANYA. I wasted my life. I'm talented, smart, brave... If I'd had a normal life I could have been someone... a Schopenhauer, or a Dostoevsky... oh my God, I'm being ridiculous! I'm losing my mind. Mama. Mama. I'm in despair. I'm dying, Mama. Help me!

(He runs to his **MOTHER**. *She embraces him.)*

MARIA. Sweetheart. Pull yourself together.

VANYA. Mama! Tell me what to do. No, wait, don't tell me. I know what I have to do. *(Looking at the* **PROFESSOR**.*)* You're going to remember me!

*(***VANYA*** leaves. ***MARIA*** follows him.)*

MARIA. I'll talk to him.

(She exits.)

PROFESSOR. People, what the hell is going on here? Keep that madman away from me. We can't live under the same roof – his room is right next to mine! He can move to town, or out to the barn. I won't stay in this house with him...

YELENA. We have to get out of this house today. Somebody needs to make the arrangements.

PROFESSOR. He's a nobody! A nothing!

SONYA. *(Fighting back tears.)* Have some compassion, Dad! Uncle Vanya and I are so unhappy! Show us some compassion! You remember when you were just starting out, Uncle Vanya and Grandma spent every night editing your papers... night after night! Uncle Vanya and I have worked so hard for you, we were afraid to spend a single penny on ourselves, we sent everything to you. You really got your money's worth from us! I don't mean that – I'm not making sense. But please try to understand how we feel, Dad. Show us some compassion.

YELENA. Alexander for God's sake go talk to him. Please.

PROFESSOR. Fine, I'll talk to him. *(Beat.)* I'm not accusing him of anything, I'm not angry, but you have to admit his behavior is weird. To say the least. But, fine, I'll go talk to him, Lena, if that's what you want.

*(The **PROFESSOR** exits.)*

YELENA. Be kind to him. Try to calm him down.

*(**YELENA** follows him.)*

SONYA. Nanny! Nanny...

MARINA. It'll be all right, little one. The geese honk and honk...and then they stop.

SONYA. Nanny.

MARINA. You poor thing, you're shivering like someone left you out in the cold! Don't be sad, little orphan, God will have mercy on all of us. I'll fix you a little tea with honey. Don't cry, little orphan...

*(**MARINA**, angry, looks to the door.)*

MARINA. Shut your beaks, you stupid geese! Go to hell!

*(Offstage, a gunshot. **YELENA** is heard screaming. The **PROFESSOR** comes running in.)*

PROFESSOR. Stop him! Stop him! He's gone crazy!

*(**YELENA** and **VANYA** appear. She tries to wrestle the gun from him.)*

YELENA. Give me the gun. Give it to me right now!

VANYA. Let go of me, Lena! Let go!

*(Freeing himself, he looks around for the **PROFESSOR**.)*

Where is he? Ah, there you are!

*(He shoots at the **PROFESSOR**.)*

Bang!

(Pause.)

I missed? I missed him again? Goddammit...

*(He smashes his gun on the floor, and sits down exhausted. The **PROFESSOR** is in shock.)*

YELENA. Get me out of here – or just kill me. But I can't stay here. I can't.

VANYA. What am I doing? What am I doing?

SONYA. *(Softly.)* Nanny. Nanny.

End of Act Three

ACT FOUR

(Vanya's room. This is his bedroom and also the estate office. By the window is a large table covered with account books and a mess of other papers. Astrov's drawing materials, paints, and portfolio sit on a smaller table nearby. Somewhere in the room is a globe.)

(A quiet, autumn evening. **MARINA** *is alone with her feet up, enjoying a cocktail.* **WAFFLES** *enters.)*

WAFFLES. Marina, aren't you going to say goodbye? They're leaving in a few minutes.

MARINA. *(Re: her drink.)* Not much left.

WAFFLES. You hear they're moving back to the city?

MARINA. Mmmm that's too bad.

WAFFLES. Do you know what all of this means, Marina? I guess they're just not country people. It wasn't their destiny to live here. No one escapes his own fate...

MARINA. Whatever it means, thank God. That was a horrible scene today – everybody screaming and shooting off guns. Shame on all of them!

WAFFLES. Yes, it was really something, wasn't it? A scene worthy of Goya's paintbrush.

MARINA. I'm too old for it!

(She drinks.)

MARINA. Things can finally go back to normal. Breakfast at eight, lunch at one. We'll sit down to supper at five like decent people. Me, I'm just an ordinary sinner who wants to eat a nice bowl of noodles.

WAFFLES. It's been such a long time since we had noodles.

(Pause.)

Such a long time. *(Beat.)* This morning, I was walking through town and some guy shouted "Freeloader!" at me. *(Beat.)* It hurt my feelings.

MARINA. Don't you pay attention to them, sweetie. We're all freeloaders off of God. Besides, you work! You, Sonya, Vanya, we're all working hard, all of us! Where is Sonya?

WAFFLES. She and the doctor are looking for Vanya. They're afraid he's going to kill himself.

MARINA. Where's his gun?

WAFFLES. At the bottom of the pond. *(Whispering.)* It just slipped out of my hands.

MARINA. *(Smiling.)* Naughty boy!

(**VANYA** *enters, followed by* **ASTROV.**)

VANYA. Stop following me. *(To* **MARINA** *and* **WAFFLES.**) Go away. I'm sick of you watching over me.

WAFFLES. Of course, Vanya. Right away.

(**WAFFLES** *tiptoes out.* **MARINA** *follows.*)

MARINA. Goose! Ga-ga-ga!

(She picks up her drink and exits.)

(**VANYA** *looks at* **ASTROV.**)

VANYA. Leave me alone!

ASTROV. I'd love to. I've been trying to get out of here all day. But – I repeat – I'm not leaving until you give me back what you took from me.

VANYA. I didn't take anything from you.

ASTROV. I'm serious. Stop wasting my time.

VANYA. I didn't take anything!

ASTROV. Really? I'll wait one more minute, and then I'm sorry, I'll have to use force. We'll tie you up and search you if we have to. I'm not kidding.

VANYA. Do whatever you want.

(*Pause.*)

God I'm an idiot! I shot twice and missed him both times! I'll never forgive myself.

ASTROV. If you felt like shooting something, you should have aimed at your own head.

VANYA. It's weird. I tried to murder someone but nobody has come to arrest me. You know what that means? *You all think I'm crazy. (He laughs.)* Yeah I'm the crazy one! Not that heartless mediocrity who hides behind the title "professor" – he's not crazy! Not the woman who marries an old man and then cheats on him in front of everyone. I saw it, I saw you kiss her!

ASTROV. Yes, *sir*. I kissed her, *sir*. And here's one for you.

(*He moves to kiss* **VANYA.**)

VANYA. (*Pushing him away.*) The whole world is crazy for putting up with assholes like you.

ASTROV. You're saying stupid shit.

VANYA. Well, I'm crazy, I have the right to say stupid shit.

ASTROV. Stop it. You're not crazy, you're just a freak. A freak and a clown. I used to think there was something wrong with being a freak, that it meant you were abnormal, or sick. But now I've come to the conclusion that being a freak is the natural human condition. You're perfectly normal.

VANYA. *(Covering his face with his hand.)* I'm so ashamed. If you only knew how much shame I feel! It's this sharp, stabbing kind of pain I've never felt before. It's unbearable. What do I do? What do I do?

ASTROV. Nothing.

VANYA. Give me something! Oh my god... I have what, maybe fifteen years left to live. That's so long! How am I going to live through all of that time, how will I fill my days? *(Squeezing* **ASTROV***'s hand.)* If only I could start over... if I could wake up on some clear, quiet morning and begin a whole new life, if the past could somehow disappear, or float away like smoke. *(Weeping.)* A new life... how do I start? Tell me how to begin...

ASTROV. Oh c'mon. What new life? No new life is coming, not for us. Our situation is hopeless.

VANYA. You really believe that?

ASTROV. Yes, I do.

VANYA. Then give me something, please... *(Touching his chest.)* I feel like I'm burning up.

ASTROV. Stop it! *(Softer.)* Listen to me. If there are any humans left on Earth in a hundred years – well, first they're going hate us for having lived such stupid, selfish lives – but maybe, just maybe, they'll also have figured out a way to be happy. You and I, though...? I think the best we can hope for is that, as we lay dying, we get to see some incredible visions. *(Tenderly.)* Vanya, you and I used to be the only decent men living out here in this wasteland, but the last ten years have worn us down. Life out here has poisoned us and made us just as awful as everybody else. *(Beat.)* But you have to stop changing the subject. Give me back what you took from me.

VANYA. I didn't take anything.

ASTROV. You took a bottle of morphine out of my bag. Look, if you want to die, go out into the woods and shoot yourself. But give me back the morphine. Otherwise, people will say I gave it to you. It's bad enough I'm the one who will have to do the autopsy. Do you think that'll be fun for me?

> *(SONYA enters with the NEIGHBOR kid, who witnesses the following scene.)*

VANYA. Leave me alone!

ASTROV. Sonya, your uncle stole a bottle of morphine from my bag and he won't give it back. Tell him he's being stupid. I don't have time for this. I need to go.

SONYA. Uncle Vanya, did you take the morphine?

> *(Pause.)*

ASTROV. He took it.

SONYA. Give it back. Why are you scaring us? *(Tenderly.)* Give it back, Uncle Vanya! I'm unhappy too but I won't give in to despair. I'll bear my unhappiness and I'll keep bearing it for the rest of my life. You have to bear it too.

> *(Pause.)*

Give it back! *(Kissing his hands.)* My dear, beautiful uncle, my wonderful uncle, give it back! *(Weeping.)* You're a good man. Have some compassion for us and give it back. We have to keep going, Uncle. We have to keep going!

> *(VANYA takes the bottle of morphine from a drawer and hands it to ASTROV.)*

VANYA. Here, take it! *(To* **SONYA**.*)* But we have to start working right away, we have to start doing something, otherwise I can't. I can't...

SONYA. Yes, we'll work! As soon as we say goodbye, we'll sit down and start working.

(Looking through invoices.)

What a mess, we've let everything go.

*(***ASTROV*** puts the morphine in his bag.)*

ASTROV. Now I can finally leave. *(To* **NEIGHBOR** *kid.)* C'mon I'll give you a ride.

*(***YELENA*** enters. ***ASTROV*** pauses.)*

YELENA. Vanya? Are you here? We're leaving now. *(Beat.)* Go talk to Alexander, he has something he wants to say to you.

SONYA. Talk to him, Uncle Vanya.

(She takes his arm.)

We'll go together. You and Dad have to make peace. It's important.

*(***SONYA*** and ***VANYA*** exit. ***YELENA*** stays.)*

ASTROV. *(To* **NEIGHBOR** *kid.)* Wait for me outside.

(A beat. He nods and exits.)

YELENA. I'm leaving. *(She gives him her hand.)* Goodbye.

ASTROV. Already?

YELENA. We're all packed up.

ASTROV. Goodbye.

YELENA. You promised me you wouldn't come here anymore.

ASTROV. I remember. I'm leaving right now.

(Pause.)

Did you get scared? Is that what happened?

(He takes her hand.)

Is it really that scary?

YELENA. Yes.

ASTROV. Stay. Just stay. Come visit me tomorrow afternoon –

YELENA. No. I've decided. The only reason I'm brave enough to look you in the eye is because we're leaving. *(Beat.)* I want you to respect me.

ASTROV. *(Impatient.)* Stay! You have to stay. Admit your life is boring and sooner or later you're going to give in to your feelings. And won't it be better if it's not in some noisy city, but out here in nature? At least it's poetic... the autumn is gorgeous out here. All these forests and falling-down old farm houses, straight out of a novel...

YELENA. You're funny. I'm so mad at you...but I'm going to remember you with pleasure. You're an interesting, original person. And since we'll never see each other again, why hide anything? I went a little crazy for you. Well... Let's say goodbye as friends. No hard feelings.

ASTROV. Yeah, you should go. *(Thinking.)* You seem like a good person but there's something deeply weird about you. You and your husband showed up here, and we all dropped everything and spent the whole summer obsessed with both of you. You infected us with your idleness. I went out of my mind! I spent a whole month doing nothing – people got sick, cows got loose in my forest and ate up a bunch of my trees. Wherever you and your husband set foot, you bring total destruction. I'm joking, but still... I think if you stayed the devastation would be enormous. I'm sure I wouldn't survive it. *(Beat.)* And I don't think it would end well for you either. So yes, you should go.

(**YELENA** *takes a pencil from his desk and puts it in her pocket.*)

YELENA. I'm taking your pencil as a souvenir.

ASTROV. It's strange, we got to know each other and now we're never going to see each other again. I guess that's what life is. Could I kiss you goodbye?

(*She nods. He leans in and kisses her on the cheek.*)

Well, that was wonderful.

YELENA. I wish you all the best.

(*She looks around. She embraces him forcefully. Something happens.*)

I have to go.

ASTROV. Yes, go. Hurry up. Get out of here.

(*Enter the* **PROFESSOR, VANYA, SONYA, MARINA, WAFFLES,** *and* **MARIA** *with a book.*)

PROFESSOR. (*To* **VANYA.**) Let's let sleeping dogs lie, eh, Vanya? "He who dwells in the past shall have his eye plucked out!" After everything that's happened in these past few hours – well, I have lived through so much that I think I might have another book in me! Something for future generations about how we ought to live! I accept your apology, Vanya, and I hope you will accept mine. Goodbye!

(*They embrace.*)

VANYA. You'll receive the same amount every month just like you always have. Everything will stay the same. Everything will be just like before.

(**YELENA** *hugs* **SONYA.**)

PROFESSOR. Goodbye, dear Mama.

(The **PROFESSOR** *kisses* **MARIA**'s *hand.)*

MARIA. Oh my precious Alexander, please take a picture of yourself when you get there and send it to me. *(Hugging him.)* You know how dear you are to my heart.

WAFFLES. Safe travels, Professor! Don't forget us!

PROFESSOR. *(Kissing* **SONYA**.*)* Farewell. Farewell, ladies and gentlemen! *(Shaking* **ASTROV**'s *hand.)* Thank you for your wonderful company. I have great respect for your ideas, your way of thinking, your passion, but allow an old man to leave you with some parting advice: there is work to be done! Ladies and gentleman, there's so much more work to be done in this world!

(He bows to the group.)

I wish you all the best!

(He exits, followed by **MARIA**, **SONYA**, **WAFFLES**, *and* **MARINA**. **VANYA** *turns to* **YELENA**.*)*

VANYA. Goodbye. Forgive me. *(Beat.)* I don't think we'll ever see each other again.

YELENA. *(Moved.)* Goodbye, sweetheart.

(She kisses him on the head and exits.)

ASTROV. *(To* **VANYA**.*)* You're not going to see them off?

VANYA. I... no. I can't. I need to occupy myself with something as quickly as possible. Work. I need to work.

(Pause. Offstage, the sounds of the **PROFESSOR** *and* **YELENA** *driving away.)*

ASTROV. They're gone. The professor must be ecstatic. There's not enough gout medicine in the world to make him come back here.

*(A pause. **MARINA** enters.)*

MARINA. They're gone.

*(**SONYA** enters.)*

SONYA. They're gone. *(She wipes her eyes.)* I hope they'll be safe on the roads. *(To **VANYA**.)* Well, Uncle Vanya, let's do something.

VANYA. Let's get to work.

SONYA. It's been such a long time since we sat together at this table. *(Re: her pen.)* It's out of ink…

(She gets up to find a new pen.)

I'm sad they're gone.

*(**MARIA** enters, slowly.)*

MARIA. They're gone!

*(She putters around lost for a bit and then finds a place to sit down and read. **SONYA** sits with **VANYA** and looks through a mess of papers.)*

SONYA. Let's start with the bills. Everything's such a mess. You take this stack, I'll take the others.

*(**VANYA** starts looking through his stack.)*

VANYA. These are from last spring…

*(They both work in silence. Writing checks. Filling out invoices. **MARINA** yawns.)*

MARINA. Beddy-bye time for me…

ASTROV. It's so quiet. Pens scratching, crickets chirping. It's so warm here, so cozy. I don't want to leave.

(Pause.)

Well, my friends. Time for me to say goodbye, to all of you. And to my table. Bye-bye little table.

MARINA. Why are you in such a hurry? Sit for a while.

ASTROV. I can't.

VANYA. *(Calculating.)* Looks like we owe two hundred seventy-five from July...

(The **NEIGHBOR** *kid enters.)*

NEIGHBOR. You ready to go, doctor?

ASTROV. Ah, yeah. I'll be right there. You mind taking these out for me? *(Handing him the maps.)* Be careful – don't crush them.

NEIGHBOR. I'll be careful.

*(***NEIGHBOR** *kid exits.)*

ASTROV. Okay then...

SONYA. When will we see you again?

ASTROV. I don't know. Summer? Roads are gonna be bad this winter. Of course, if something happens, let me know – I'll find a way to get here. *(He shakes her hand.)* Thank you for the food and the company, and especially for your kindness. *(To the room.)* Thank you for...well, for everything.

(He goes to **MARINA.***)*

Bye-bye, my sunshine.

MARINA. Don't you want a little snack before you go?

ASTROV. No, ma'am.

MARINA. How 'bout a nip of vodka?

ASTROV. Ah...why not?

*(***MARINA** *exits.* **SONYA** *and* **VANYA** *continue to work. After a pause.)*

ASTROV. I lost a few more chickens last week.

VANYA. You need to put up new netting.

ASTROV. Yeah. I've been meaning to get around to it.

(*He idly spins the globe.*)

Must be so hot in the Amazon right now.

VANYA. Probably.

MARINA. (*Handing him a glass of vodka and a piece of bread.*) One for the road! To your health, sweetie.

(**ASTROV** *drinks the vodka.*)

Now eat some bread!

ASTROV. No thank you, that did the trick! So, goodbye! Don't see me off, Marina. I'm fine on my own.

(**ASTROV** *leaves.* **SONYA** *follows him.* **MARINA** *sits down in her armchair.*)

VANYA. June second… two hundred dollars… February sixteenth…

(*Pause. The sound of* **ASTROV** *driving away.*)

MARINA. He's gone.

(*Pause.* **SONYA** *re-enters.*)

SONYA. He's gone.

VANYA. That's almost a thousand bucks. Plus seven hundred from April…

MARINA. (*Yawning loudly.*) God forgive us all.

(**WAFFLES** *enters on tiptoe and quietly tunes his guitar.* **VANYA** *pets* **SONYA**'s *hair.*)

VANYA. Oh sweetheart. Everything feels so heavy tonight.

SONYA. I know but what can we do? We have to live.

(Pause.)

We will live, Uncle Vanya. We'll live through a long row of days and quiet evenings, and we'll be patient with whatever life sends our way. We'll keep working and working, and when our time comes, we'll die, and there, beyond the grave, we'll say that we suffered and that we cried and that life was hard, and God will have mercy on us. And you and I, Uncle, my dear Uncle, you and I will see a bright new life opening up before us, a beautiful life, filled with grace. We'll look back at our past unhappiness with tenderness, maybe even with a smile – and we'll rest. I believe it, Uncle. I believe it with all my heart.

(She embraces him.)

We'll rest!

*(**WAFFLES** quietly plays the guitar.)*

We'll rest! We'll hear angels, we'll see the sky lit up like diamonds, we'll see our suffering drowned in mercy, a divine mercy that rains blessings on the entire world. Life will become gentle, sweet, and tender as a kiss. I believe it, I believe it... *(Wiping his tears.)* Poor Uncle Vanya, you're crying. You've never known real happiness but you wait, Uncle Vanya, you wait... We will rest... *(Holding on to him.)* We'll rest!

*(**WAFFLES** plays softly. **MARIA** knits or prays her rosary. **MARINA** writes on the margin of a pamphlet.)*

We'll rest.

End of Play

www.ingramcontent.com/pod-product-compliance
Lightning Source LLC
Chambersburg PA
CBHW070649120726
47909CB00004B/1639